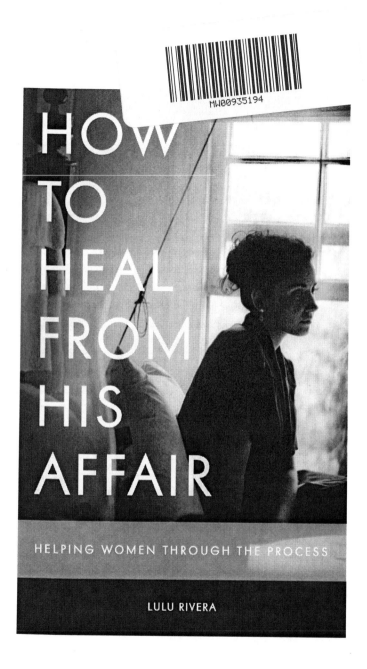

HOW TO HEAL FROM HIS AFFAIR

HELPING WOMEN THROUGH THE PROCESS

LULU RIVERA

First Edition

ISBN-13: 9781974481828 (Paperback)
ISBN-10: 1974481824 (Electronic Book)

Library of Congress Control Number: 2017914298
CreateSpace Independent Publishing Platform, North Charleston, SC

Visit the author's website at www.lulurivera.com.

Table of Contents

Dedication

To my sister, my best friend, my counselor, and my cheerleader, Nilsa Rosario. You are a wounded healer who never stops helping others. You have always been my rock, my role model, and my mentor. I love you more than you will ever know. THANK YOU FOR EVERYTHING!

Alone in the Process

Many people are familiar with the ministry called "Proverbs 31 Ministries" and its founder, Lysa TerKeurst. On June 13, 2017, she bravely announced that she was divorcing her husband of 25 years due to his infidelity. I would see people posting her material on Facebook so I was familiar with the ministry name. When I read her announcement, I could relate to her experience and her pain. Unless you have walked in her shoes, you cannot understand the difficulty of being a ministry leader and making the decision to end a long-term marriage. She said, "God has now revealed to me that I have done all I can do and I must release him to the Savior."

When I began writing this book, I was still married to my first husband and I had chosen to stay married to him after he committed adultery.

However, he committed adultery again and things got worse so we ultimately divorced. Like Lysa, I tried both options, reconciliation and divorce, during my 20-year marriage.

There are many books written to help couples who have experienced adultery to move toward restoration. I read several of these books. There were a few problems with the ones I read. The Christian ones were intended to be read and followed by couples who are serving God together. Well, so much for that! I was the only one serving God in the relationship. The secular ones, were aimed at the couple seeking reconciliation. How was I to move forward without my husband partnering with me in the process the way the books mentioned? I just had to do it alone. Others were too spiritual, almost to the point of being unrealistic. Yet other books were so clinical they were boring. I believe that's why it took me so long to heal and move forward.

I didn't have a lot of proper guidance in the healing process. I had my sister in the East Coast that I would talk to by phone but I hated bombarding her with all my problems. I didn't have any family nearby that I could go to for refuge. My pastors at the time did not know how to help me. A few of my friends tried to encourage me. Others told me to dump him! Yet others just stayed away from me while I went through this ordeal. Even my therapist didn't help me much. As a woman who had never married, she could not relate to my issues. She was just somebody I could vent to for a fee! During my years at the King's University, I met two ladies through my online classes who gave me wise counsel. This is when my healing process began.

If you're reading this book, chances are you are suffering from the effects of your husband's betrayal and you may feel alone in the storm. I encourage you to seek healing and restoration for yourself as a person and not just for your marriage. You don't have to be alone in the healing process if your husband doesn't join you. You're too valuable to allow this crisis to cripple you or destroy you.

May the grace and power of God carry you through this journey so that you can move forward toward restoration and wholeness. Don't give up. There is hope.

Chapter 1
A Distress Call

Have you ever felt so much pain in your heart that you could hardly pray? Have you cried out to God so much that you wondered if He even hears your prayers? Psalm 6 shows us that King David experienced some of that. In Psalm 6:2-3 it says, "Have mercy on me, O Lord, for I am weak; O Lord, heal me, for my bones are troubled. My soul also is greatly troubled; But You, O Lord—how long?" When I discovered my ex-husband was committing adultery, the pain was so immense that I would attempt to pray but all I did was wail. I felt as if God had forgotten me because I felt no relief from the pain. I felt perhaps I did something to deserve this pain. I felt so weak and helpless.

King David knew what it felt like to feel tremendous distress and to wait on God for deliverance. In verses 6 and 7 it says, "I am weary with my groaning; all night I make my bed swim; I drench my couch with my tears. My eye wastes away because of grief." These verses described me during that long and horrible period in my life. I cried every night and hardly slept. I thought my life was over. It was difficult to face another day with all that pain still in my heart. I became weary. My soul was distressed. I thought God took a vacation during my darkest hour. I kept calling on God to deliver me from this anguish. Verse 9 tells us that the Lord does hear our supplication; He receives our prayers. He hears our weeping.

We live in a fallen world where people have a free will. Sometimes those people choose to sin against us. It is not always because we did anything to deserve it. It is because they decided to make selfish decisions. Even though we go through times of darkness, the Word of God reminds us that He is near to us. His grace is what carries us through those dark times. You should never feel alone because you're not. Know that God does love you. But you must endure until the end. It may seem hopeless but it is not. God knows just how much you can bear before your breaking point. In the end, you come out stronger than ever and able to help others in their times of darkness.

Answer the questions that follow each chapter in this book or keep a journal of your healing journey. Keep track every day of your emotions, your night dreams, and your thoughts. This will help you see if you are progressing or if you get stuck somewhere in the healing process.

Reflect:

- What emotions are you feeling today?

- Have you prayed about it?

- Who have you talked to about it?

- Write down all the questions you have.

- Make a list of what you want God to help you do, get through, accomplish, and/or deal with today.

Chapter 2
Is Healing Possible?

You just discovered your husband is having an affair. Your mind is overloaded with thoughts. Your emotions are hard to control. You feel like you're dreaming because there's no way this could be happening to you. Confusion hinders you from taking the proper action. What should you do? Should you beat the hell out of him? His mistress? Should you kick him out?

When I discovered a love letter from the mistress to my ex, I began shaking. I didn't know what to do. That letter confirmed what I suspected for over a year. Every time I questioned him about the different clues I found, he always had explanations. I had that horrible gut feeling that he was being unfaithful but didn't have hard evidence. After finding the letter, I panicked trying to figure out how to handle the situation. Since he had gone somewhere, I packed a diaper bag, grabbed my 10-month-old baby, and drove to my pastor's house. Before I left my home, I placed the love letter on the desk in the office so that when he returned he could see that I knew about his infidelity.

Shortly after kicking him out, he managed to convince me he was sorry and that he loved me and wanted to stay married to me. Being super emotional and distraught, I believed him and allowed him to come back immediately. After all, we had been married at that point for ten years and had just given birth to our first child. This was the beginning of a roller coaster of events.

It was extremely difficult to find healing after having been deceived, lied to, and cheated on for many years. He lied excessively and deceived me so much that I just didn't know what to believe anymore. It felt like my brain was hurting from mental anguish. His affair with this woman lasted about three years that I know of. It began when I conceived my first child. It ended months after I gave birth to my second child.

When the affair finally ended, I had to find healing for myself and I eventually started trusting him again. I believed him when he said he'd never put himself through that again. Just when I felt I was making progress, he began a second affair. History repeated itself. Although I didn't have solid evidence, I found clues throughout the first four years of their affair.

Many women ask if they can survive their husband's treachery. The answer is yes, but it is not easy and it is a process. Do all women recover? We all know at least one person in life who never recovered from the loss of a relationship or never forgave someone who betrayed them. We should never allow another human being to have that kind of power over us. We can either be constructive or destructive over the loss we have experienced. Which do you choose? Victim or victor?

I read a letter online that was written to Dr. David Hawkins, a marriage therapist. The female writer wrote the following about the healing process after adultery, "This is the most difficult process I've ever been through." She ended the letter by saying, "We are healthier now than ever before." There are couples who heal from the infidelity and manage to make the marriage work. Some of the women I interviewed testified to that. However, many others end in divorce.

To make the marriage work, both spouses must work together toward that goal. The relationship will never work if only one spouse does all the trying, which is the dilemma many women experience. The husband must be willing to make many changes after he's had an affair. The wife must be willing to move forward without repeatedly reminding him of what he did. This can be difficult for some women, especially when the pain has been so severe. The unfaithful man must be remorseful about his actions. Remorse is different from an apology. He must also be willing to deal with the consequences that result from adultery.

A betrayed woman will probably need a lot of time to be able to "trust" again; the man must be willing to accept that. Many men will not want to wait around for this to happen even though they are the ones who cheated on the wife. The man must be willing to stay accountable to his wife. Men will see this as being on a "leash" or as having no privacy. Again, they forget it was their actions that led to this place of distrust.

It is "privacy" that opens a huge door to adultery. Nowadays it is very easy for someone to have their own email address and their own cell phone. No longer does the mistress need to call the house telephone like they did in the old days. This makes it so easy for people to commit adultery because their spouse may not have passwords to their cell phones and other accounts. In my case, my ex would give me the password and then change it! If you constantly ask for the password, your spouse will try and make you feel guilty for not "trusting" him. That way you can back off and he can carry on with his secret life. I was made to feel bad and was accused of being suspicious and not trusting.

In the chapter titled, "Preventing Adultery," I list all the things a couple ought to abide by to prevent adultery. If a man wants to make his marriage work again, he should be willing to comply by the list. He must sever ALL ties with the lover even if it means moving, getting another job, changing his cell phone number, cancelling his email address, etc. Whatever it takes!

A wife will need time to heal. The husband may say, "I already said I'm sorry, so get over it and move on." What people fail to realize is that healing is a process, sometimes a really long one. Some experts say that it will take the woman the same length of time the affair lasted in order to heal. For example, if the affair lasted 3 years, the woman may need about 3 years to heal. For those who have a hard time forgiving (like I did), it will take longer.

The severity of the affair will also affect how long it takes the wife to heal. For example, if the husband had just a one-night affair, then the wife is more apt to heal quicker from it than an affair in which the husband carried on a whole separate life with the mistress (which was the case with me). If the husband had an affair with a woman who was friends with his wife, that can be even more difficult to heal from because of the betrayal by both parties. It is a double whammy. There are some affairs in which the husband did everything except live with the mistress. Perhaps the husband left his wife for a time to live with the mistress and then returned to his wife only to continue the affair secretly (my case again).

You might ask at this point why a man would return to his wife if he's not happy in the marriage only to continue the affair. Some therapists say that a man will stay in the unhappy marriage because of familiarity. He knows what to expect in the marriage. But to start over with another person would be risky because he would not know what to expect. I heard a preacher once say that we begin to dishonor (family members) as familiarity sets in. This is what happens in a marriage.

It is important you rely on the Holy Spirit to do a work of restoration in you. God can restore you, your husband and your marriage only when BOTH are willing. It is essential that you pray God delivers your husband and restore him first unto God and then unto yourself. Renew your mind daily with the Word of God. Encourage yourself even when it is hard to do so. If you can't encourage yourself, find somebody trustworthy that can encourage you. Do not feel you must go through this alone. Sadly, some people will not always be there for you when you need them. Therefore, learn to encourage yourself.

Not all marriages are restored no matter how much you pray. Did I just shatter your theology? Let's just keep it real! Some people are just dead set in their ways and are NOT willing to do whatever it takes to make their marriage work. These people remain in the marriage for selfish reasons. For almost 20 years, I prayed every prayer there was and it still did not cause any change in my husband. I read self-help books, prayed, fasted, decreed, declared, bound and loosed, cancelled curses, rebuked Satan and demons, and put anointing oil on his pillow. He did not change. The adultery continued. He also displayed contempt toward me.

I finally had to make the decision to walk away from a marriage that I believed was dead and from a husband that continued to mistreat, disrespect, dishonor, and betray me. There is plenty of evidence to prove that I made the right decision.

People sometimes get stuck in a stage in life where hurt was experienced. If that happens, they will continue to live life in an unhealthy manner. When people are not honest with themselves and do not admit that they have unresolved issues, it just leads to defeat. My ex had issues that he refused to confront. That seems to be the case for many women I've interviewed. Their husbands were also dealing with unhealthy issues but refused to get help. At that point, a woman must decide to either stay in the unhealthy, destructive marriage and be a martyr or leave and be healthy for her and her children.

When I finally chose to leave the marriage, a tremendous sense of liberation came over me. I felt like chains were broken off. I became spiritually revived. A veil of deception was lifted. I experienced God in some powerful ways. There are things we do not see when we are in the midst of a storm. Sometimes we are in denial because we don't want to believe our spouse is really doing this to us or that our marriage is coming to an end. Therefore, we choose to ignore the red flags, the clues, or the knot in the stomach. We want to give the spouse the benefit of the doubt.

Eventually God blessed me with a husband that treats me far better than any man I've ever met. It is mind blowing how perfect we are for each other. He honors me and treats me with respect. He is an open book. There are no secrets, no hidden passwords, NO PORN, no meetings with women, and no unresolved issues! He is a God-fearing man whose heart is in the right place. I now have peace like I never had before. Since starting a new chapter in my life, my ministry has grown and God has used me in many ways. My husband and I have so much in common; same convictions, same worldview, and same desires. Joyce Meyer once said, "What happened in my life may not have been Plan A, but God can take Plan B and make it better than Plan A ever would have been."

Reflect:

- What emotions are you feeling today?
- Does your husband have any unresolved issues from the past? Have you ever discussed them?

- Do you have any unresolved issues? List them.

- Does your husband have a relationship with God?

Chapter 3
Emotions and Defenses

Extreme emotional pain is very dangerous. Please seek help as soon as you feel you are at the verge of a breakdown. Many women have tragically taken their lives and/or the lives of others because they had a moment of hopelessness or temporary insanity because of their pain.

On July 13, 2017, Jessica Edens murdered her estranged husband's alleged mistress in Greenville, SC. She then drove to Easley, SC, parked her car at a speedway and shot to death her four-year-old daughter, her nine-year-old son, and herself in the head. For a woman to kill her own children is a clear indication that she lost her mind at that moment. People do not consider how their betrayal will affect the betrayed person or even others. Some people cannot handle the pain of adultery, separation, and/or divorce.

There were times when I felt I was about to lose my mind and did things I now regret. One day while pregnant, I got in my car with my baby in the back seat and began driving fast and erratically toward nowhere in particular. In that moment, I called my sister in New York and told her what I was doing. She graciously talked me into pulling over somewhere. She listened to me as I cried. She talked to me until I finally calmed down and realized I was putting myself and my child in danger.

There are many different emotions you may experience when you discover the adultery, even after it has ended. You may also build up a few defense mechanisms. Defenses are given to us by God to help us deal with suffering. However, they are meant to be temporary. We are never to stay stuck in any of these areas. Otherwise, they turn into strongholds.

Most people have heard the acronym DABDA. This represents the five stages of grief: Denial, anger, bargaining, depression, and acceptance. These stages usually occur in that order but not always. Sometimes people move to one stage and then revert to a previous stage.

The first emotion experienced is **shock** or **denial** or both. It is almost impossible to believe that the man you married, the man you love could betray you. For a Christian, it's worse because you feel embarrassed or ashamed. Your life is supposed to be an example to others. You may believe that having God in your life is supposed to exempt you from suffering. Well, it doesn't! Nobody is exempt from temptation and suffering. But having God in your life makes all the difference in having hope for the future and becoming whole again.

Once you have accepted the fact that your spouse has cheated on you, you may feel tremendous **anger**, **betrayal**, **rejection**, and **abandonment**. You begin to feel **numbness** and **confusion** because you don't know what to do. **Fear** then sets in; you may think he'll leave you for the other woman. You may fear that your family is about to be torn apart. If he already left you, you fear being alone the rest of your life. You may ask yourself, "How can I make it without him?" All sorts of irrational fears begin to grip you.

Some emotions are difficult to control. Anger is a very strong emotion, which all the women I interviewed admitted experiencing. They felt angry at themselves, angry it happened to them, and later angry at their spouse. You too may feel angry at your husband for what he did to you or angry at yourself. You may feel angry at the mistress! In my case, I was angry I didn't do more to expose my ex's affair to get him and his mistress into trouble. I had the thoughts but never followed through. I was angry that because I was a Christian I chickened out. Although I did do some things that got them into trouble. Try to get a hold of your anger and not do anything you will later regret. Be angry but sin not (Ephesians 4:26)!

Some women may get angry at God for allowing it to happen. What we need to understand is that each of us has a free will. God cannot hold anyone back from doing what he or she wants to do. James 1:14-15 says, "But each one is <u>tempted</u> when he is drawn away by his <u>own</u> desires and enticed. Then, when desire has conceived, it gives birth to sin; and sin, when it is full-grown, brings forth death."

At times, you may feel you're about to go insane. So many unreasonable thoughts may run through your mind. You may even want to do some things you thought you'd never do. You may have already done some! One time, my ex and I were having a very heated argument over his affair. Since he had threatened to take my children from me, I somehow thought that if I cut my arm up, I could tell the police he did it to me. I figured if I can't have my kids, neither can he. Talk about irrational thoughts! I never thought my actions could be used against me because the police would think I'm a danger to my kids! Well, he called the police on me because I began to hit him on the chest. When the police arrived, they inspected me for bruises and they saw the cuts on my arm. They were not deep cuts, just superficial scrapes. But God in His grace toward me allowed a female cop to come along with two other male officers. She felt compassion toward me when I broke down and told her he was having an affair. She had just experienced something similar in her personal life. She advised me to "dump the loser!" They asked my ex to leave our house that evening and they did not report the incident.

Hatred and **bitterness** can build up in your heart because of the hurt he caused you. What many women do is hate the mistress more than they hate their spouse as if the spouse had little to do with the adultery or were pressured into it. Seriously? Ladies, he had as much to do with it as did the mistress!

Anxiety and **desperation** can occur if he's still having the affair or if you're separated. You become anxious about what's going to happen to you, your kids (if you have any), the marriage, and whether he still loves you. You become desperate for answers and for ways to win him back. You have no peace during this stage.

You may want to take matters into your own hands. You may even get tempted to cheat on him. Don't do it! Here is where you need to believe that God will vindicate you. Just don't ask God when and how! It will be in His time, not yours. Romans 12:19 says, Beloved, do not avenge yourselves, but rather give place to wrath; for it is written, " vengeance is Mine, I will repay, says the Lord." Be careful not to get caught up waiting for God to vindicate you. It indicates you are still holding onto bitterness. We all reap what we sow. Job 4:8 says, "Even as I have seen, they that plow iniquity, and sow wickedness, reap the same."

After we got back together, I began to feel bitterness and disgust toward my ex. I became indifferent toward him. It's as if the reality finally hit me of what he did to me. I think what I was doing was subconsciously paying him back for the hell he put me through. I became cold and unloving. It took about two years before I realized I wasn't healed yet and began changing my attitude and actions toward him.

You may begin **bargaining** with your spouse, begging him to come back (if he left you). You'll beg him to give the marriage another try. You'll beg God to bring him back. Ladies, let's have some dignity here. It's okay to let him know you want to make the marriage work but there's no need to humiliate yourself. This can work against you. Some men see it as weakness. It can empower them. If you must beg a man to love you and be with you, then he is NOT the man for you even if he is your husband! There is such a thing as marrying the wrong person. Some examples in the Bible are: Abigail and Nabal, and Samson and Delilah. Being unequally yoked comes with a price.

The opposite of begging can also happen. Some women may become defensive to protect themselves from any more pain. They end up pushing the spouse further away.

Stonewalling can occur on your part or both. Dr. John Gottman, a relationship researcher, was the first to apply this term to couples. It is defined as, "when a listener withdraws from an interaction by getting quiet or shutting down." The term may remind you of Stonewall Jackson. He got his nickname because he stood like a stone wall during a war. During stonewalling, there won't be any communication. Nothing will get resolved. Both parties grow cold toward each other.

Depression and **sadness** are very common emotions. Depression is extreme sadness. In the case of adultery, it may be a result of unresolved anger. It will take time to work through it. Never rush to a doctor to get on anti-depressants. You'll only make matters worse for yourself. Take the natural and safe way toward healing. Keep an eye on the sadness so as not to allow it to last too long, otherwise, it will hinder your healing. Even worse, it can lead to hopelessness, which produces suicidal thoughts, like what happened to Jessica Edens.

You should NEVER feel that the only way out of your problem is suicide. You are way too valuable to God. Remind yourself that you are not alone. There are many women experiencing the same thing as you. Psalm 30:5 says that weeping may endure for a night, but joy comes in the morning. I think the psalmist was referring to a night in the Arctic Circle where night lasts for months! Of course, I'm being facetious. But really your healing is up to you.

Shame is another emotion you may experience. As a Christian, and as a church leader, I felt ashamed that my spouse had cheated on me. We were supposed to be role models. This is not supposed to happen to church leaders, right? Sadly, it happens way more than we realize. I felt I had no business ministering to others because of the mess I was in. There were times I felt ashamed that I divorced while being a Christian. I felt like I now had a blemish on my ministerial role.

Low self-esteem comes when a woman asks herself, "Was I not pretty enough?" Or, "What is wrong with me that my husband had to run to another woman?" Some women go to the gym and start working out, they run to the plastic surgeon and have enhancements done, and/or they visit all the stores to buy a new wardrobe. I know women who did all of the above! However, usually appearance is not the primary reason why men cheat. In Chapter Four, I discuss reasons men commit adultery.

The emotion of **grief** will eventually set in. You will grieve the loss of trust, loss of intimacy, and whatever else you have lost in the marriage. I remember breaking down crying a few years after the adultery. I was still grieving the loss of many things that died in my marriage. Grief is natural and necessary so don't rush it and don't suppress it. If people around you are advising you to hurry up and heal and move on, then kindly remove them from your life until you have gone through the grief process. Nobody can rush through grief. In fact, years later you may find yourself breaking down in the oddest places or at the strangest times and it will be due to grief.

Resentment may creep in. This is when you begin to feel indignant toward your spouse because of the sin he committed against you. You realize that he did you wrong and you become angry or bitter toward him. This is what happened to me after the first affair. As I mentioned earlier, I became cold and indifferent toward my ex because I kept reminding myself of all the pain he caused me. Obviously, when you're feeling resentful you cannot move forward in reconciliation because resentment is a form of vengeance.

It's okay to experience these emotions and defenses. It is all part of the healing process. You cannot heal from something that you don't acknowledge. Accept that you're feeling these things and then deal with it. Do not, however, allow yourself to get stuck in any of these emotions and defenses for a long period of time. Defense mechanisms can help carry you through severe pain, but be aware that these are reactions that happen to help you avoid more pain.

Similarities among the betrayed women

While interviewing survivors of adultery, I discovered that the women all believed they had a happy marriage (including me). Most of them did not personally know the mistress. They all had a personal relationship with God. They felt used. They felt like fools. One lady, Jodie, went into depression and gained weight. It took her ten years before she decided to seek counseling. She remained married and is now experiencing a happy marriage.

Another lady, Lydia, experienced low self-esteem, questioning what was wrong with her. The affair occurred nine years after being married. She blamed herself for not being good enough. She gave the marriage a second chance and it lasted nine more years. Sadly, her husband had another affair. That's when Lydia chose to divorce her spouse. God then blessed Lydia with an awesome, successful, and God-fearing man who was everything she needed and wanted.

Life is not over when you experience adultery. We never know what the outcome will be. We just have to believe it will all work out in our favor in the end. The important thing is to hold on to God with all your being while going through the journey. If you truly rely on God, trust Him, and believe His Word, then it will work out for you.

If you don't already exercise, this is a good time to begin doing some form of physical activity. It really helps the mind and body. I took up jogging during this season and it really helped me feel better about myself. I used that time to talk to God, worship Him, reflect, and clear my mind from negative thinking. I strongly recommend that you develop a lifestyle of worship. I have felt God's presence many times during my worship time. The Bible says He gives perfect peace to those whose mind is stayed on him.

Reflect:

- What emotions or defenses are you experiencing?

- How do you express your emotions?

- Where are you in the grief process?

- Do you have a support system? (Family, friends, a church?)

- If you belong to a church, are they equipped to help you?

- Are you praying daily even if it is just groaning?

Chapter 4
Reasons Men Commit Adultery

Let's be honest here, does the reason why men cheat really matter when your heart has been run over by an 18-wheeler (figuratively)? Nevertheless, since some women are curious why, I will mention a few.

Many people go into a marriage with baggage. That baggage entails unresolved issues. Some of those issues may be:

- Low self-esteem
- Inferiority
- Low self-worth
- Sexual abuse
- Addiction to pornography
- Family curses
- Distrust/suspicion due to past relationships

- Distorted thinking

These unresolved issues carry over into the marriage thus causing problems to arise. If a man feels low self-esteem, he will continue to seek approval from women. This is why couples should seek pre-marital counseling before they say, "I do." Important issues can be dealt with before the marriage vows are taken. Honesty is crucial from the beginning of a relationship.

If you search the internet, you will find hundreds of secular articles on the top-ten reasons why men cheat. Everybody, from *Psychology Today* to *Cosmopolitan*, has their own list of reasons. In the past, however, research showed that the primary reason men cheated was because of unmet needs. While "unmet needs" is still in the top-ten list of reasons, there are other reasons given as #1. It depends whose list you consider credible.

When men feel underappreciated they look elsewhere for validation. Some men want their wives to be kind and thoughtful not nagging and pointing out their flaws. Yet other reasons are:

- They want to get out of their marriage
- Lack of sex in their marriage
- They don't love their spouse anymore

- They feel acceptance by other women
- They want to prove they still "got it"
- Easy access to the opposite sex
- Money and power
- Peer pressure
- Porn
- Loneliness
- Dissatisfaction
- Narcissism
- Culturally accepted behavior

Spiritually, however, the reasons men commit adultery are:

- They lack an intimate relationship with God; their minds are not regenerated
- Do not fear the penalties of their sins
- Sexual perversion (lust of the flesh and eyes)
- Lack of self-control; no self-discipline
- Family curses
- Depraved minds

If your husband works in an environment where adultery is commonplace and he is weak in that area, chances are high he'll commit adultery. We all know that adultery is rampant in the entertainment and music industry. In my case, my ex started working in a certain law enforcement agency where adultery was commonplace (I'm not claiming in any way that all cops are cheaters, this just happened to be the case in the department my ex worked in).

Since my ex already had it in him to be unfaithful and was needy, it was the perfect environment for him to commit adultery again. One time he had the audacity to tell me, "All this time I was beating myself up for having had an affair and it turns out all the cops do it!" Can you imagine how my blood pressure rose at that moment? So, guess what happened? He had another affair. He would use the excuse that he had to sleep at the jail or at the police station because of his hours. This time it was harder for me to jump in my car and go stake him out. I never knew where he was.

My ex met his second long-term mistress in the jail he worked at since she too was a cop. They began an affair rather quickly and she filed for divorce from her husband four months after she began her affair with my ex. I remember finding an invoice in my ex-spouse's papers. It was for her divorce from her then husband. I questioned him as to why that paper would even be among his belongings. I also asked who she was. He said that paper must've been put in his mailbox at work by mistake. You probably want to ask me, "You actually believed that crappy lie?" Yes, I did, even though it sounded very strange that a personal document like that would have been placed in her mailbox at a police department. This happened at the very beginning of him starting out in law enforcement and to be very honest, I did not think he would commit adultery again. Therefore, I gave him the benefit of the doubt.

The devil has successfully managed to convince most men in our society to get involved in pornography. So many men watch porn because they believe it is normal for all men to do it. One time my ex justified doing porn and masturbation because he heard a famous rapper say on national television that he masturbates to porn several times a week even though he is happily married. Even though not ALL men do it, the numbers are high. No longer do men need to pay to look at porn. It is so readily available and it's free! The problem is that it leads to other forms of perversion not just adultery. To make matters worse, there are many women willing to post nude pictures and videos of themselves on the internet.

Our culture is full of self-absorbed, narcissistic people who enjoy posting selfies on social media. The more provocative the pictures, the more attention they get. Our society truly has deteriorated. It is clear by looking at all forms of media that our society has hardly any role models of women who are moral, classy, have dignity, and self-respect.

If your spouse is addicted to porn, he will become curious or driven to act out what he is viewing in private. In pornography or sexual addiction, there are levels. The more it is viewed, the more he wants. Pictures or videos are no longer enough and the viewer wants to take it to another level. That level is to partake in an extramarital affair. It could then lead to having multiple partners at the same time. It can also lead to experimenting with same-sex partners and group sex. It is never ending until the person acknowledges it is a problem and it is morally wrong.

It has become easy to be unfaithful. The internet, cellular phones, and social networks have made it very easy for people to connect privately. If you have spent a night at a hotel, then you've noticed how porn is readily available on the hotel's television. In fact, according to an article I found on blogs.thegospelcoalition.org dated April 10, 2015, Jared Wilson stated that a hotel manager said that the youth pastors conference attendees staying at his hotel broke the record for the most porn viewing than all previous conferences. This indicates that porn addiction is just as prevalent in the church as it is among unbelievers and it must be addressed in the church.

Here's another thing about adultery: it's not just physical. You can have an emotional affair with someone you have not had sex with. Many men think they can masturbate while watching a woman strip live via streaming and do not consider it adultery.

I mentioned earlier that married couples are withholding passwords from each other because they have been convinced that we all need some privacy! Each spouse has his and her own email address, cell phone, and even computer. Is it really necessary to have everything separate?

If the suspicious wife asks for passwords or to see his accounts, the husband will become hostile and say, "I'm sick of you not trusting me!" Or he might say, "can't anybody have some privacy without being drilled?" So, the suspicious wife will feel guilt for questioning her husband and she'll back off. Ladies, if you have a gut feeling he's having an affair, keep digging because you will find what you're looking for! If you're the type of person that is overly suspicious and doesn't trust because of past issues then I say back off. But if your spouse has shown many indications that he is having an affair and you're sick to your stomach, then more than likely you are correct.

Our society is becoming increasingly immoral. Marriage is becoming less sacred. People don't respect the fact that someone is married. They will keep pursuing that person anyway. They don't fear the consequences of infidelity or of going to hell. Bottom line is that adultery is a result of selfishness! (James 1:14-15.)

Reflect:

- Have you blamed yourself for the affair? If so, why?

- Has your husband given you an excuse for the affair? If so, how do you feel about it?

- Has your husband taken responsibility for his actions?

- Is there anything you want to do that you feel would improve yourself or the marriage? (For example: Stop nagging him, stop having fits of anger, or communicate better.)

Chapter 5
Reconciliation Versus Divorce

One day I was reading the Spirit Filled Life Bible by Jack Hayford. I was reading I Corinthians Chapter 7. By the way, this passage refers to when someone leaves you for reasons other than adultery. As I read verse 11 where it says, "But even if she does depart, let her remain unmarried or be reconciled to her husband. And a husband is not to divorce his wife." The word, "reconcile" stood out to me. I read the Word Wealth section in the Bible where it explained the definition of the word, "reconciled." It was defined as, "To change, exchange, reestablish, restore, relationships, make things right, remove as enmity." It also said that this word, "describes the reestablishing of a proper, loving, interpersonal relationship, which has been broken or disrupted." At this point, I realized that my marriage had never been reconciled.

Just because you get back together with your spouse doesn't mean reconciliation has occurred. My ex continued to breach the marital contract even after I chose to stay with him and give him another chance. Four years into the second affair, I found a love letter from her to him. He had no intentions to dump the mistress. She was content being the part-time lover. I can guarantee that the three-fold cord Ecclesiastes 4:12 is talking about does NOT refer to a mistress in the midst of your marriage! I realized the best thing to do for me and my children was to divorce. My children were really being affected by the animosity between their dad and me. It was horrific and very painful.

Unfortunately, today, a huge number of married couples experience the pain of adultery. Many studies show that it is mostly men who commit adultery. However, women are catching up. There's also no difference in numbers for those claiming to be Christians. Regardless of who commits the act, both spouses must make the painful and difficult decision to either reconcile or just get a divorce.

Reconciliation can be painful because of the constant reminder of how your spouse betrayed you. Moreover, you live in partial fear that he will do it again. Remember, if your spouse was in love with his mistress, it will be very difficult for him to get over that love. Love is a very powerful emotion. Furthermore, sexual intercourse creates a soul tie that can be very difficult to destroy. It will take extreme actions on his part to never contact his mistress again. Reconciliation with you will not take place until he has completely lost his love for his mistress. Are you willing to wait?

Is it better to get a divorce? It all depends who you ask and on the individual's situation. In my case, I chose to try again. Although there might exist many similarities, each relationship is different because people are different. Biblically, a woman has the right to divorce a husband who has committed sexual immorality or if the husband walks away from the marriage (Matthew 5:32 and I Corinthians 7:15). We always hear that God hates divorce. But God hates infidelity even more. In Jeremiah 3:8 we read that God divorced Israel due to adultery.

Some couples may choose separation instead of divorce. I learned in my research that

70 percent of couples that separate end up in divorce. There are three reasons why this may happen:

1. It allows the betrayer to spend more time with the mistress, thus causing that relationship to grow and yours to diminish.
2. One or both spouses realize they can survive without the other.
3. One or both realize they no longer want to be in that marriage. Therefore, be prepared should the outcome be divorce.

The separation period should be used to develop a friendship with your spouse, not to date others. You can develop boundaries during this time. This is a time to heal and reflect on the future. It is recommended that there be no sex during this period. I'm not sure how realistic that is!

Does God prefer reconciliation? Yes, but reconciliation can only work IF there has been genuine repentance and forgiveness and both parties are willing to do their part. Both spouses need to love, respect, and honor each other.

In my first marriage, I felt my ex's love for me was never restored. He treated me harshly. He would tell me to shut the "f..." up or get the "f... out of my face." He was verbally and mentally abusive. He had no respect for me. He would argue with me frequently, curse at me, and the list goes on. I continued in the marriage anyway still hoping one day he would change and treat me right. It never happened. In fact, he continued doing all the things he did during his first affair but worse. I had strong suspicions he was having another affair but needed hard evidence even though I had found things that were questionable or inappropriate. The second time around, he perfected the infidelity. He covered his tracks very well. As I mentioned earlier, since he was a police officer, my ex used that as an excuse for the supposed long hours at work and not coming home.

One day I found myself sinking further into depression. I felt I was spiraling down into a pit. I was miserable, extremely unhappy, and worse yet, I didn't know how to get out of it. I kept praying for God to remove my ex out of my life because I thought I wasn't supposed to be the one to leave the marriage since I was a Christian. This kind of distorted thinking keeps many women in bondage. I had every right to divorce him. I finally made the decision to separate after 20 years or marriage.

Many women have asked me the tough question, "should I stay with him or should I get a divorce." Before answering that question, you should write down several things on paper. Write the <u>reasons</u> why you should stay together and why you should get a divorce. Write down what you stand to gain or lose if you divorce. Write down what may have been the reasons that led to the adultery. Then if you choose reconciliation, seek immediate counseling (either together or alone) to discuss the problems that existed before the adultery. The decision to divorce should never be made in haste. It is one that should be done after much thought and prayer, and with a heart free of vengeance.

There are several common reasons why couples stay together. One reason is because they still love each other even though their needs are not being met. However, sometimes love is not enough. Another very common reason is because of their children. Is that a good enough reason if the affair is still ongoing and you both continue to fight? Is it a healthy decision? Some experts say that a toxic marriage is more damaging to children than a divorce.

As I mentioned previously, one reason why the cheating spouse will stay married is that familiarity is better than the unknown. The spouse already knows what to expect in the existing marriage even if it is a bad one. To leave the familiar can be a bit scary and a bit risky. Besides, what if it doesn't work out with the mistress? The husband can always fall back on the wife if the wife allows herself to be used in this manner.

Here are other reasons women tend to stay in a failing marriage:

- They still love their husband and still hope things will change even though he's had several affairs.
- They are afraid to be on their own.
- They cannot imagine losing their home, the comfortable or secure lifestyle, or having to work full-time outside the home.
- They feel that all men are alike and if they get a divorce, the next man will also cheat on them so they might as well stay in the failed marriage.
- They are in denial and refuse to believe anything's wrong in the marriage.
- They believe it is the Christian thing to do.

- In some cultures, or religions, the woman never divorces her husband no matter what.
- Some women stay because of the history they share together.

I chose to stay in my marriage for the following reasons:

- I believed that God hates divorce. In Matthew 19:8, Jesus said to the Pharisees concerning divorce, "Moses, because of the hardness of your hearts, allowed you to divorce your wives, but from the beginning it has not been so." It was never (and still isn't) God's will for people to divorce.
- I believed God would intervene.
- I believed God would turn my marriage around thus giving me a testimony to share with others. The problem with this is that my ex had a free will and God cannot do anything if He is not given permission to do so. My ex had to be willing to serve God and allow God to be in the center of the marriage. That did not happen.
- Since we had a baby and a toddler I did not want our family ripped apart.

- I did not want to give the enemy, Satan, pleasure in knowing he destroyed another marriage. In the book, "Sacred Marriage," Gary Thomas says, "Don't abort your history with the spouse whom God has called you to love." So, I chose to stay but at what cost? If anything, my ex was the one who aborted our history because of his sexual appetite and lack of control. Many times, we blame Satan for everything but all he can do is send an agent on assignment to tempt you because of your lack of self-control (1 Cor. 7:5). It is up to you to resist the devil and he will flee, but only if you submit to God.

Many women think about how it seems easier for a man to move on and marry another woman. Some men will purposely make the second marriage work and avoid the mistakes they made in the first marriage. They do in the second marriage what they should've done in the first one. Some will start a new family, have kids with the new wife and develop a closer relationship with the new kids. They will be there for the new kids because they didn't do it the first time around. He already made all his mistakes with the first wife and has gotten all his foolishness out of his system. The husband is now older, more mature and probably ready to genuinely settle down. I have seen this happen to many people. I didn't want that to happen to me. I didn't want another woman to end up benefitting from all my pain. It didn't seem fair. My thinking was, "I might as well give my husband a second chance and allow him the opportunity to make up for all the mistakes he made." Your spouse must want to stay and make it work because he still loves you, is remorseful, and is ready to stop being unfaithful. That was not the case with me.

It is possible to stay together and make it work. Jim Tolle, former Pastor of Church on the Way in Van Nuys, California once said he saw Christ in his wife because of how she chose to treat him after he committed adultery. That statement really made me think. I realized I had done the opposite (during his first affair). I had not chosen to forgive and extend grace to my then husband. An evangelist I saw on television once said that when he committed adultery, his wife said to him, "I will never bring it up if you don't bring it up." Neither one ever brought it up again and had a beautiful marriage after that. There was genuine repentance and forgiveness, and they were willing to make it work.

Divorce changes people's lives forever. It is compared to death. Therefore, it is important to really make a well thought-out, prayerful decision. Both spouses must be willing to make it work. Otherwise, if it is only you who wants to keep trying, then get ready to keep hurting and suffering. But if divorce is the best remedy, then move forward with it. I personally hate divorce and what it does to families. I strongly believe in reconciliation and forgiveness. But I also know that sometimes adultery can destroy a family beyond repair.

To those of you who are asking, "should I stay or should I go?" Only YOU can answer that. I hope you will consider carefully the circumstances and the ramifications of divorce. Also consider the effects of staying in a bad marriage. If you choose to stay, I suggest you seek wise counsel first. Dr. Tim Clinton says in his book, *Before a Bad Goodbye*, "The greatest marital tragedy can be overcome, and God can take the bad and use it for His good." He goes on to say, "Your marriage can be rebuilt; it can be more beautiful and exciting than ever before. How? By following God's plans for love and life."

If your spouse does not want to do his part, you should do what is best for you and your children. Nobody can be forced to do something against his/her will. You should also be aware of the risk of becoming infected with a sexually transmitted infection or disease.

Divorce should never be chosen to vindicate against your spouse. Many women rush to get a divorce because their husband cheated. They are doing it as a way of saying, "I'll teach you a lesson; now you're going to lose me forever!" Well, that doesn't always work. There's no need for us to vindicate ourselves. Sin punishes the sinner. Proverbs 6:28-29 says, "Or can one walk on hot coals, and his feet not be scorched? So is he who goes in to his neighbor`s wife. Whoever touches her will not be unpunished."

Those who commit adultery will face the consequences sooner or later. You don't need to hope and pray that your husband burn in hell (as tempting as it is)! Your goal should be to seek healing, peace and restoration. When your husband sees that you are not vindictive, he will realize what a tremendous woman he has or had and your actions may cause him to regret what he did. Otherwise, he will feel justified in having cheated on you and he will feel tempted to do it again if you stay together.

I know couples who jumped the gun and got a divorce based on how they felt at that moment without really thinking things through and they regretted it in the long run. I also know some couples who kept trying and trying and still got divorced in the end. And then there are those couples who not only survived the horror of adultery but are now happier than ever. The important thing is that you try.

If you choose reconciliation, it is important you perform an evaluation. That evaluation should include:

- Is your spouse completely remorseful for what he did?
- Has your spouse evaluated himself? Does he understand what is broken in him? Is he willing to get help and fix it?
- Is your spouse willing to deal with the consequences that result from his betrayal?
- Does your husband have any legitimate complaints about you that you are willing to work on?
- Are you ready to put behind you his infidelity and not bring it up continuously?

- If something triggers the betrayal incident, how will you both handle the emotions that it will produce?
- Have you asked your husband all the questions you wanted answers to regarding his affair? Knowing all the details can hurt you even more.
- Do you both understand that it will take time to heal and trust again?

The "F" Word

You cannot write a book about healing and not mention the subject of FORGIVENESS! That dreaded "F" word that nobody likes to hear when they are in agony. This is a subject that should not be dealt with too early in the healing process. A woman should not be forced to forgive too early because it can affect her later. A woman needs time to deal with her emotions, her thoughts, and her decisions. However, it does have to be discussed because it can hinder healing.

A woman never forgets the memories of the betrayal. If it was a very painful time, any little thing will stimulate a woman's memories. Thus, she will relive those awful times and start hating her husband all over again! That is why the woman must seek God with all her heart. A woman cannot do it in her own strength. She must CHOOSE to forgive her husband WHEN she's ready to forgive. Notice the key word is "WHEN." Too many times people are forced to forgive before they are ready. This can cause resentment and/or anger in the victim. Once she's ready to forgive, she should do so daily until she knows without a doubt that she has truly released him to God. Why? For two reasons: Firstly, forgiveness is a process. Secondly, because it's easy to fall back into the bitterness, anger, and unforgiveness.

How do you forgive your husband after all he's done to you? There are tons of books available about forgiveness so I will not get into details. What I will discuss is what worked for me and what worked for the women I interviewed on the subject. I confessed every day out loud the words, "*Lord, I choose to forgive my husband. I choose not to vindicate for what he's done to me. Lord, I release my anger, hurt, pain, bitterness and hate toward my husband. Replace those feelings with love, compassion, and forgiveness.*" I prayed this continually for a long time. I also prayed for his salvation because I wanted my kids to have a Godly father.

Catch yourself when you begin to entertain memories from the past. Those memories will cause you to relapse in your forgiveness process. You must reject those thoughts. Otherwise, it will bring back the destructive emotions you've been working so hard to overcome. If people bring up anything that stimulates your negative feelings from that season in your life, either tell them to change the subject because you will not entertain it, or avoid them altogether. I chose to leave behind me most of the people I knew during that time (mutual friends and neighbors). If you have mutual friends who choose to remain "neutral" and choose not to bring correction to your spouse, then they don't need to be in your life.

I do have to interject one thing here about forgiveness. You should not tell someone you have forgiven them if they never repented. They will look at you and think you're crazy. As shocking as it is, some people don't acknowledge that they've sinned against you. If you read the scriptures, you will see that God did not forgive anyone who did not first repent. Moreover, Jesus said in Luke 17:3, "Take heed to yourselves. If your brother sins against you, rebuke him; and IF he repents, forgive him."

If your spouse has not repented, you ask God to prepare your heart for when he's ready to ask for your forgiveness. You release your spouse to God and release all your negative feelings to Him as well. A good book to read about biblical forgiveness is *Rediscovering the Power of Repentance and Forgiveness* by Dr. Leah Coulter. Some people will never repent because of their pride.

"How do I know I have forgiven him?" If you still wish he would get run over by a truck then chances are you have not forgiven him! If you still get upset every time you think about what he did and colorful words come out of your mouth, you haven't forgiven him. If you still talk bad about him, you haven't forgiven him. There are times when we need to talk about what happened and then there are times we need to keep quiet because it doesn't benefit anyone. If after 20 years you still throw it in your spouse's face, you seriously need counseling! If your spouse has done his part to reconcile with you, make up for what he did, and is a great spouse now, then throw that issue into the sea, the way God throws your sins into sea after you repent.

H. Norman Wright gives some great advice in his book, *Recovering from the Losses of Life*. There, he wrote a chapter titled "The Loss of a Relationship." In it, he advises to write a letter to your spouse. Put all your feelings in it. On one side of the paper, you write what you forgive him for. On the other side, you write whatever comes to your mind that contradicts what you forgive him for. For example, if you say, "I forgive you for cheating on me." Across from that, you write something like, "I hate you for leaving me." I did a letter like this one. I never gave the letter to my ex because it was only for therapeutic purposes. I read the letter over and over out loud until it no longer affected me or made me break down and cry. That was when I knew I was beginning to heal and release him. I then ripped up the letter and threw it away. This was very effective for me.

Reflect:

- What are the reasons you would choose to stay in your marriage?

- Is your husband willing to stay married?

- Are you both willing to get counseling?

- If your spouse doesn't want counseling, are you willing to get it for yourself?

- Are you the type that holds on to offenses?

- Are you ready to release your spouse (and all he has done to you) to God?

Chapter 6
Domestic Violence

Abuse comes in different forms. In many cases, the adulterer is also abusive toward the wife in one or more of the following ways:

- Physically
- Verbally
- Emotionally
- Spiritually
- Economically
- Nonverbally
- Sexually

The act of domestic violence has increased recently to epic proportions. Many women are uneducated on this subject and, therefore, allow the abuse. The Violence Against Women Act is a federal law that was enacted in 1994 and has been revised several times. This law provides programs and services to female victims.

According to the National Coalition Against Domestic Violence, 1 in 3 women have been physically abused by an intimate partner. Physical violence against a woman by a spouse or intimate partner is a criminal act. This means that domestic violence is now treated as a serious crime instead of just a private matter. It also means the abuser can be sentenced to prison. Does this law solve all the domestic violence problems? Absolutely not. You must get to the root of the problem to change the behavior.

There are men who believe they did not physically abuse a woman because they did not slap or punch her. Yet according to the American Academy of Experts in Traumatic Stress, physical abuse includes the following:

- Pushing, throwing, kicking
- Slapping, grabbing, hitting, punching, beating, tripping, battering, bruising, choking, shaking
- Pinching, biting
- Holding, restraining, confinement
- Breaking bones
- Assault with a weapon such as a knife or gun

- Burning
- Murder

Here are some reasons why men abuse women:

- They have rage and don't know how to control themselves.
- They want to control the victim.
- They are under the influence of drugs and/or alcohol.
- It's part of their culture.
- Learned behavior - They watched their mom be abused or they were abused.
- Economic hardship (extreme poverty).
- They are demon possessed.
- They are psychotic.

Many women fail to call the police during the abuse for several reasons:

- The victim thinks she deserves the abuse.
- Fear that the abuser will become even more aggressive.
- The victim doesn't want her partner to go to jail because the abuser is her only source of income.
- In some states, the abuser can be sentenced to jail and the victim is not allowed to drop the charges.

- The victim is an illegal immigrant and thinks she will be deported back to her country if she reports it. This thinking is quite common among Hispanic immigrants. The law makes exceptions to abused parents of a U.S. Citizen or if the immigrant wife is married to a lawful permanent resident. For more information on this subject, refer to www.uscis.gov. There are other exceptions listed on the website under the Form I-360. The information is also available in Spanish.

In an article in Time Magazine dated February 27, 2013 titled, "What's Wrong with the Violence Against Women Act?" the author stated, "VAWA has increased prosecution rates of domestic violence cases, but there is little conclusive evidence that it has significantly reduced the incidence of violence." Domestic violence continues to be prevalent, especially in certain geographic areas and in certain cultures.

An article I found on the postandcourier.com website dated September 19, 2016, listed the top five states ranked as the deadliest for women in domestic abuse:

- Alaska

- Louisiana
- Nevada
- Oklahoma
- South Carolina

Here's the terrifying part, almost everyone you meet in South Carolina (where I live) attends church every Sunday. Yet we rank in the top five states in domestic abuse! This indicates that churches are filled with wife beaters! It takes more than laws to change a person. Individuals can only be changed by the power of God. Abusers need to be delivered from the strongholds that cause them to commit these unthinkable acts against women. Then they need to be transformed by the renewing of the mind as stated in Romans 12:2. Imagine if churches cared just as much about the abused women as they do about people paying tithes. I have nothing against paying tithes; I believe in giving. However, tithing seems to take precedence over people's healing, deliverance and transformation.

On the greenvillesc.gov website for the Greenville Police Department, it states, "On average, according to the National Domestic Violence Hotline, a victim will leave an abusive relationship seven times before leaving for good." This is a sad statistic.

It is crucial that a victim learn what her rights are, what the law says, and that she needs to leave that relationship immediately. The victim will also face a long road to recovery and healing from the emotional and psychological results of the abuse. No woman ever deserves to be abused!

There are many resources available to victims. Perform an internet search in your area and you will find them. To some people, it sounds crazy that a victim would want to return to an abuser but many women do. The only way you should ever consider going back to an abuser is if there is clear evidence that he has been completely set free, has changed his behavior, is involved in some form of accountability group, and is still attending therapy sessions.

A powerful book on this subject, which I recommend is *Broken Children, Grown-up Pain* by Paul Hegstrom, Ph.D.

Reflect:

- Have you experienced any of the forms of abuse listed in this chapter? If so, how often? Have you ever dealt with it together or alone?

- Do you know any women experiencing abuse? If so, encourage them to leave that situation immediately and assist her in finding help.

- If you belong to a church community, is your church equipped to assist victims of domestic violence? If not, encourage them to do so.

Chapter 7
Preventing Adultery

Although this book is written with the intentions of helping women go through the healing process, it is beneficial to add a chapter on how to prevent adultery. Even though adultery has already occurred, many couples continue to make the same mistakes that allowed the door to be open to the temptation of committing adultery.

One common statement made by someone who committed adultery is that it wasn't planned, "it just happened." Adultery doesn't just happen. There are steps that are taken by two people who desire to be together. The way in which a husband and wife can prevent falling into the trap of adultery is by taking preventive steps. The following list may seem absurd or overwhelming to some people but when you're trying to save your marriage, you will do whatever it takes!

- A big mistake is when a person says, "I would never do that." Never assume you are so righteous or self-controlled that you could never do such a thing. Instead, you need to think it can happen to you.

- If your needs are going unmet, you need to tell your spouse. Get marital counseling or a marriage coach. Otherwise, it is almost sure you will end up having an affair.

- Conduct yourself properly at all times in an upright manner.

- The second you find yourself thinking a person is attractive, run like hell. Do everything you can to NOT be around that person, especially alone.

- Watch what you say and do because there are consequences to your actions. Words can be misconstrued or even taken out of context. Actions can be misinterpreted. Don't flirt with someone other than your spouse. That sends a clear message that you are not happy in your marriage.

- If you are hanging around with too many singles, chances are you will be tempted to cheat on your spouse. Try to avoid hanging out with singles or with people that are having affairs. Hang out with married couples, especially ones that have a good marriage.

- It is okay to have acquaintances of the opposite sex. However, men should not have female friends that they hang out with. Likewise, women should not be hanging out with other men. Your best friend should be your spouse, not the girl/guy next door or at the job.

- Do not ride alone with the opposite sex in a car (especially when that person is attractive), and definitely not at night.

- Intimacy occurs when two people spend a lot of time together and share each other's problems and secrets. Do not tell your problems to someone of the opposite sex (especially an attractive one). This creates intimacy, which always leads to other things. Never share marital problems with the hottie at your job.

- Do not accept greeting cards or gifts from someone you find attractive or someone you think is attracted to you.

- Wear your wedding ring. Although nowadays people rarely care that you are married, it is still a good idea to wear it.

- Think "consequences." What if I do this thing, will my spouse be bothered by it? Will my marriage be affected by it?

- If you attend school, as many adults do now, do not study with someone of the opposite sex. Men need to find a man to study with or to call for information. Women need to find another woman.

- Do not hug or kiss the (attractive) opposite sex. This is too risky.

- Do not allow the opposite sex to visit your home if you are alone.

- Respect and honor your spouse. Do not belittle, mock, curse, be sarcastic, call names, accuse falsely, physically hit, yell at, deceive and lie to one another. Do not put down your spouse in public (or private). It causes shame, embarrassment and low self-esteem. Do not take your spouse for granted.

- If your spouse asks you to disconnect yourself from a certain person, you ought to respect their wishes and do so. It has nothing to do with them trying to control you. It has to do with them perceiving a potential threat.

- Be accountable to your spouse and to a trusted friend. Do not complain that you feel like you have no privacy. Privacy is what leads people to have affairs. Be an open book. With today's technology, every person has their own cell phone and their own computer. This opens a tremendous door for a spouse to cheat because of the "privacy" they have. Let your spouse know all the passwords to everything you have.

This list may sound a bit harsh and it goes against the grain but it will set guidelines to help prevent you and your spouse from committing adultery. Keep open communication with your spouse. Always be willing to share what bothers you. Always keep trying to make the marriage better. Always look for ways to keep the marriage fresh.

Whenever respect, honor and kindness begin to disappear, that is a red flag that the marriage is in trouble. Start talking to your spouse and try to figure out what has gone wrong. This way it can be repaired before it gets to the point of adultery and/or divorce.

Reflect:

- Have you both discussed this list thoroughly?

- Are there any conditions you would add to this list? Any there any you would remove?

- Have you both agreed you will abide by these conditions?

Chapter 8
Do Not Grow Weary

There were times when I stopped praying because the pain was so severe; words just would not come out of my mouth. I would just wail. It reminded me of Hannah from the Book of I Samuel Chapter One. Verse 10 says Hannah had grief in her soul and wept bitterly. Oh, that was me alright. Verse 13 says Hannah prayed in her heart. Eli the priest saw how she would move her lips but no sound would come out of her mouth. Therefore, he thought she was drunk. She responded by saying, "No, my lord, I am a woman whose spirit is broken with sorrow: I have not taken wine or strong drink, but I have been opening my heart before the Lord."

Many times, I felt God was nowhere to be found because He was allowing me to suffer so much. I was angry that I had been such a faithful wife and a faithful Christian and yet God allowed this to happen to me. This can be a time where you really question your faith, whether God really does exist, what's the purpose of having faith, and what more can you possibly pray if nothing changes? Does prayer really work? We are quick to blame God and/or doubt our faith.

Here are several reasons why we experience suffering.

- We live in a fallen world.
- It can be consequences to decisions we have made; it is self-inflicted.
- Suffering can cause people to change the direction they're going in.
- It can serve as a learning experience that will prepare you for ministry.
- It can be an opportunity for God to manifest Himself in your life, for Him to intervene in your situation and bring glory to Himself.
- Suffering can also serve as a wake-up call for some people. Let us also remember that the thief (Satan) comes to steal, kill, and destroy (John 10:10).

Regardless of the circumstances, believe that God is working things out for you even though you cannot see it yet. Run to God in the same manner that the woman with the issue of blood ran after Jesus. Don't let go of God the same way Jacob didn't let go of God when he was wrestling with Him. He refused to let go until God blessed him. Have the determination that Job had when he said, "Though He slay me, yet will I trust Him." (Job 13:15)

I keep reiterating that you should seek wise counsel either through your church, a trained counselor or a licensed therapist. If your husband is still having an affair, you may want to get counseling alone. If your husband is still lying that he's having an affair, he is certainly not going to open up to a counselor and admit it. My ex met with a male counselor on his own but rarely told me anything about his sessions. That was because he was still having the affair and was strongly considering leaving me and starting a new life with the mistress. I found this out afterwards from both him and his lover. Yes, his mistress and I had a few long conversations. She threw him under the bus (as the saying goes) once she discovered he was lying to her all along.

You will need friends that are willing to help you go through the healing process without telling you that you're crazy for staying with your husband. You need people who will not judge or criticize your decision to stay in the marriage. However, if you're being warned about his abuse, take heed. You need women who are stronger than you to encourage you, lift you up, pray with you and not just say they'll keep you in prayer. You need friends that will check up on you frequently and see how you're holding up. You need friends who are discerning enough to know when to just listen to you pour your heart out and not feel they should speak a word. Sometimes you may just want someone you can cry with.

I applaud any woman who decides to hang in there and give the marriage a second chance. If you don't do it for yourself, then at least do it for your children (if you have any). I'm not telling you to stay in the marriage only for the children because it will not work. I'm saying at least try for their sake. There is nothing wrong with giving your marriage a second chance. It just might work out. If it doesn't, at least you know in your heart you did everything you can to make it work. You don't have to wonder what could have happened if you had stayed and tried again.

You will be rewarded for your faithfulness. Galatians 6:9 says, "And let us not grow weary while doing good, for in due season we shall reap if we do not lose heart." The word "weary" in

Greek means to be utterly spiritless, to be wearied out; exhausted. I believe this scripture doesn't just refer to doing good deeds. I believe it also refers to standing strong amid adversity. It means not giving in to vengeance or temptations that you will later regret. It means standing firm, immovable, and blameless. Seasons don't last forever!

As I mentioned earlier, take up some form of exercise. Never turn to alcohol or medication to drown out your sorrows. Do something that can benefit you. Talk to God throughout the day. Start your day reading the Bible, even if it is just one scripture.

In time, you will heal and dwell less on the painful memories of the betrayal. When those memories resurface, be sure not to entertain them. The enemy always tries to remind you of your painful past but it's up to you to reject it or accept it.

Reflect:

- Where are you in the healing process?

- Do you trust God to carry you through this season?

- Are you spending time with God?

- Are you journaling everything you're going through? If not, try it. It is very therapeutic.

- Set small goals for yourself.

Chapter 9
Choosing Divorce

If you choose divorce due to adultery or being abandoned, then you should not feel any guilt over your decision. Divorce is not the unpardonable sin. Remember that the Bible allows divorce when either of those two incidents occur. In fact, divorce may be the best thing that could ever happen to you. Is it possible God is allowing you a way out of something that is bad for you? Many women insist on forcing a relationship to work. They don't realize that the man could be sent by the enemy to destroy them.

Earlier I said that you should not consider divorce hastily based on your current emotions. Consider it only after you have prayed, sought wise counsel, and weighed all the reasons why reconciliation is not an option.

Divorce does not bring closure to the pain that your spouse has caused you. Divorce just merely makes it official that you are no longer bound to that person legally. You will go from being a partner in a relationship to playing both roles of mother and father if you have kids. If children are involved, then you will have to deal with your ex until the kids reach 18 years old. You will have to see his face during special occasions involving your children. The pain may resurface when your ex-spouse ends up staying with the mistress. The anger may continue until healing occurs.

Be mindful of your children. They will each be affected differently by the divorce and all the changes. Some kids become angry and start acting out. Others deal with the pain quietly. It is important you get them help if you see signs of depression or other behavioral changes.

You will have to decide if you want to keep the same friends you and your ex-spouse shared. Quite honestly, this is a good time to get rid of friends that you know will take information about you to your ex. Now you will see who your true friends are.

Divorce also brings a change in finances and in your lifestyle. You may be forced to get a full-time job if child support and alimony are not enough to take care of you and your kids. With a full-time job comes child care and other expenses.

Another change that comes with divorce is that you become the head of household. You will now oversee things your husband used to take care of such as home repairs, car issues, managing the finances (if he did that), etc.

All these changes can become overwhelming at times. You will need a support system. Make sure you have people you can talk to and assist you with different things. Get familiar with what resources are available to you as a single parent. There will be times you become sad because you're grieving the death of your marriage and that's normal. Change is part of life. It is not always easy but you must learn how to handle change so that you can move forward. Keep an eye on your stress levels. Too much stress can produce physical illnesses. Whenever I need cheering up, I watch old comedy classic movies and eat chocolate! How do you cheer yourself up?

The Divorce Process

Now is not the time to be confused. You need to be mentally stable so that you can think rationally and make good decisions that you will not regret. It is never a good idea to say hastily, "You can keep it all. I don't care." You will care afterwards and regret it! Here's a list of some things you will need to do:

- Decide if you will file for divorce on your own or if you will hire an attorney. If you don't have money for an attorney and you don't have a lot of assets, consider using a paralegal. All states are different so find out what your state allows. In California, I was able to use a paralegal. I went to the court and filed for the divorce.

- Will you have complete custody of the children? Will it be 50/50? Will it be 80/20?

- Decide how much child support you need to care for your children. My paralegal had advised me on how much to request. My ex agreed. Child support is NOT taxable income and, therefore, you do not have to report it.

- Decide how much alimony you will need. This is separate from child support. Alimony must be reported as income and you will have to pay taxes on it. Once you remarry, you will lose it.

- Will you stay where you reside or will you move? If you own a house, you will have to decide if you will sell it and split the profit or if you will keep the house as part of the settlement.

- You will need to create a Marital Settlement Agreement. This agreement will list everything that pertains to the divorce: Custody, visiting hours, the dividing of the assets (cars, real estate, money, furniture, etc.), child support, alimony, medical/dental insurance, etc.

- Who will pay for the children's health insurance?

- Make a list of all accounts that have both your names and change each one (i.e. checking accounts, credit cards, utilities, etc.). You cannot remove your name on any loan, therefore, your name will remain on it until the loan is paid in full.

- If you have both of your names on a mortgage loan, you cannot be removed from it. You can only transfer your portion of ownership of the home by filing a quitclaim deed.

So, what do you do now? Throw yourself before the Lord. Cry out to God to help you through the process of releasing anger, bitterness, and revenge. Verbalize each wrong you want to release your ex-spouse for. Repeat this as long as it takes for you to let go. *"I choose to release _____ (ex-spouse) for all the lies, for all the deception, for disrespecting and dishonoring me. I cancel his debt to me. Help me, Father, to stay free of unforgiveness, bitterness, hatred, and anger. I put it all in Your hands. In Jesus' name, Amen."*

Just because unpleasant things happen to you doesn't mean you must remain a victim. Change your perspective, trust and believe that God will work it out and bless you. You may experience a temporary setback. Your finances might suffer until you get back on your feet. You may have to move, get a new job, or even file for bankruptcy! So what! It's a new season, a new chapter and with God's help and guidance, your life can be better than it ever was. It is ALL up to you! Just make sure you have a support system that can help you through this entire season. Be positive.

Reflect:

- Are you feeling drained or overwhelmed? Do something that will take your mind off things.

- Do you have somebody that can walk through this divorce process with you? Lean on them. Do not reject any help from those that care about you.

- Have you done research on the issues you need more information on?

- Examine yourself. Where are you in the healing process?

- How can you flip this experience and make it positive?

- Are there goals you never accomplished that you can now pursue?

- Have you learned any lessons from all this?

Chapter 10
You Will Survive

We all go through difficult times in our lives. It is inevitable. The important thing is making it through those times victoriously even if it is a bad situation like adultery or divorce. The goal for you now is to be healthy and whole. You have a calling and a purpose. Experiencing pain and loss should never stop you from moving forward and fulfilling your purpose. In fact, it should propel you forward! You owe it to yourself to seek healing and to be restored as a person. The scripture that can help you to see things positively is Romans 8:28, which says, "And we know that all things work together for good to those who love God, to those who are the called according to His purpose."

Crises have a way of bringing us closer to God. We experience God like no other way. It also makes us stronger. It prepares us for life and for ministry. We can only take somebody as far as we have gone. Experiencing pain will allow us to relate to and reach out to others who are hurting. The greatest characters in the Bible had their share of crises. They were ultimately used by God in a tremendous way.

Choose to never feel sorry for yourself when you're experiencing pain and suffering. Never give up on yourself or on God. Continue to push through until you get your breakthrough. It will come! Now is a good time to create healthy boundaries between you and others. Begin new healthy habits. Step out of your comfort zone and try new things.

When you begin dating again, be careful you don't make the next person pay for the sins your ex committed against you. It is not fair to that person. It also reveals that you have not yet healed from the betrayal. Make sure you communicate what your expectations are to the new person in your life.

There's a great organization that helps people who are going through divorce. It is called Divorce Care. Their website is: www.divorcecare.org. They offer resources, care groups, articles, and daily devotionals. Another care program that is available is the Fresh Start/Life After Divorce program. You can do a web search to see if this program is available in your area. If not, perhaps, you can ask the church you attend to start one. I'm sure there are other resources and programs out there as well but you will have to do some searching.

Be encouraged; you are important to God. He has a plan for you. Know that there truly is life after divorce and it could be better than you ever imagined. Be patient during the healing and restoration process. Pray about every decision you need to make and seek wise counsel. Accomplish goals you did not have an opportunity to pursue before.

I offer free short-term Biblical counseling. For more information, my website is www.friendswithpurpose.com.

Reflect:

- Have you created a budget that you can live on?

- Have you considered joining a support group? If so, which one? How long is it? Do they charge a fee? Do they provide childcare?

- Have you started to make new friends?

- What are your short-term goals?

- What are your long-term goals?

Chapter 11
About the Author

Mary (Lulu) Rivera is a Biblical Counselor, Bible Teacher, a Life Purpose Coach, a Financial Coach and an author. She holds a Bachelor of Theology in Biblical Counseling from the King's University (Van Nuys, CA). She received her coaching training through Dr. Brazelton at the Life Purpose Coaching Centers, Int'l. Mrs. Rivera has written numerous articles, which can be found on www.ezinearticles.com. She is also the author of the book, ***Purposed for Womanhood: Walking in Your God-Ordained Role.***

The author grew up in the Bronx (New York) with her mother and two sisters. At 18 years old, she left the Bronx and attended Farmingdale University, where she received an Associate in Applied Science. Lulu gave her life to the Lord in 1987. After courting for a year a man she met in church, she married him in 1989. In 1990, she moved to California. That is where she experienced highs and lows. She was blessed to give birth to two boys. She owned her own business, pursued higher education, and flipped homes. But during those 20 years, she suffered being married to a man that lived a secret life. Throughout both pregnancies, her ex-husband was involved in long-term affairs. It was a very lonely, painful, and difficult time, especially because she was a church leader.

Like many other women, Lulu was taught you must stay married no matter what. She prayed, fasted, decreed, declared, anointed everything, and read just about every marriage book. Nothing worked. Lulu then realized that she cannot make her marriage work by herself. It takes both parties and he didn't want the marriage anymore. God will never force anybody to change. She knew she had the Biblical right to divorce her unfaithful husband. After struggling for 20 years with her husband's sexual immorality, lies, deception, and emotional abuse, she divorced him in 2009.

In 2012, she married Pastor Sam Rivera. She and her husband have the marriage they only dreamed of having. They teach, counsel, empower, and encourage many people. They have a ministry called Heartland Ministry in which they license, ordain, train, mentor and counsel leaders. God is good! Divorce is not the unpardonable sin. God has a marvelous way of restoring broken people and broken hearts, and using them to bless others.

Articles written by Mary can be found at: http://ezinearticles.com/expert/Mary_L._River a/208691. To join our group on Facebook, please search for "Friends With Purpose" and request to join.

If you have any questions, comments, or testimonies, please feel free to connect with me through email at:

friendswithpurpose@yahoo.com.

You can also visit my websites at:

www.friendswithpurpose.com or www.lulurivera.com and send me a message. Oh by the way, please leave a kind book review. Thank you!

<u>*Notes*</u>

<u>*Notes*</u>

CPSIA information can be obtained
at www.ICGtesting.com
Printed in the USA
LVOW10s1406290118
564430LV00015B/241/P